Jobs People Do

Doctors

by Emily Raij

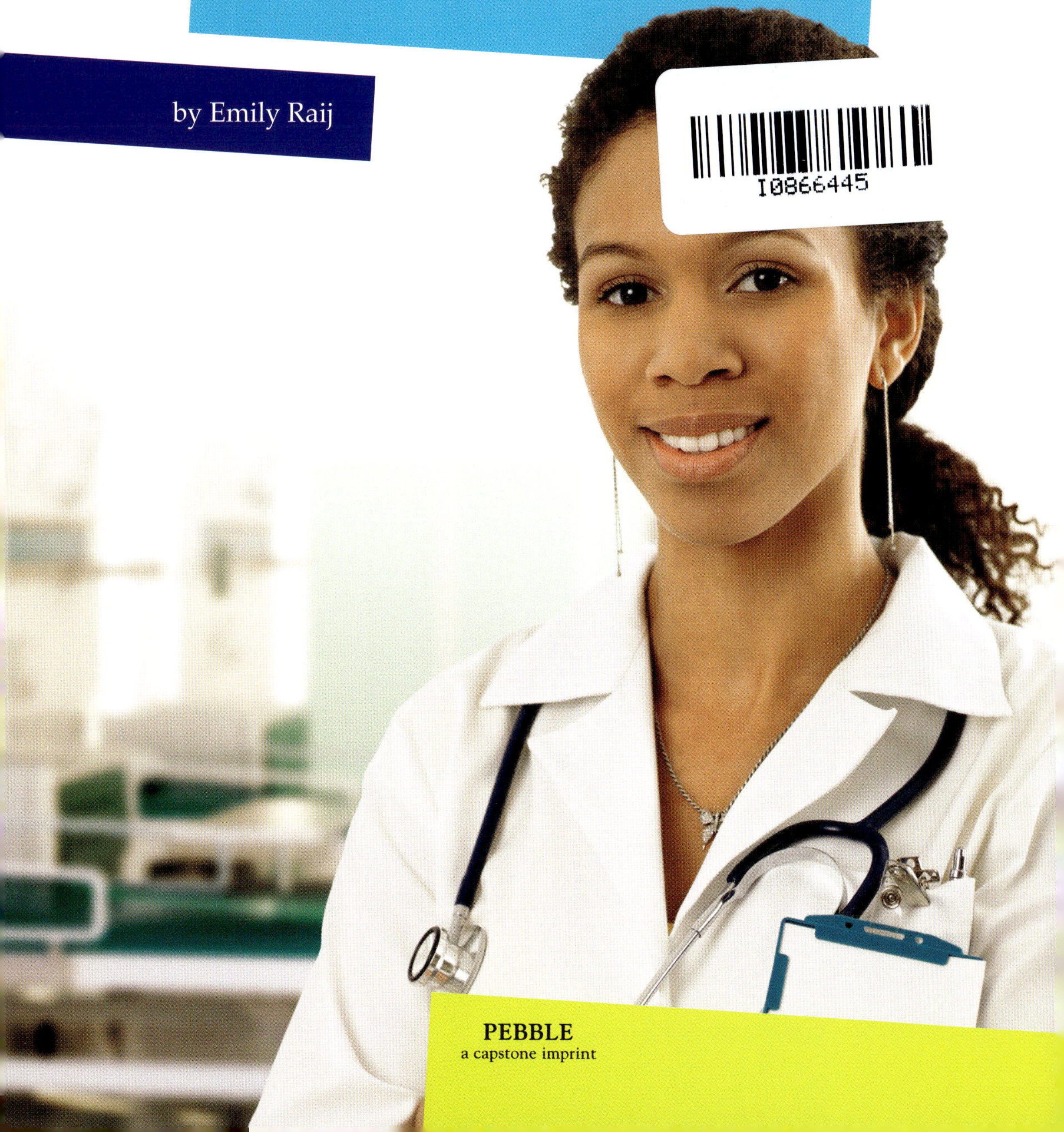

PEBBLE
a capstone imprint

Pebble Explore is published by Pebble, an imprint of Capstone.
1710 Roe Crest Drive
North Mankato, Minnesota 56003
www.capstonepub.com

Library of Congress Cataloging-in-Publication Data is available on the Library of Congress website.
ISBN: 978-1-9771-1374-0 (library binding)
ISBN: 978-1-9771-1809-7 (paperback)
ISBN: 978-1-9771-1382-5 (eBook PDF)

Summary: Learn all the roles doctors have, the tools they use, and how people get this exciting, fast-paced job.

Image Credits
Shutterstock: Andrey_Popov, 14, antoniodiaz, 27, ARTFULLY PHOTOGRAPHER, 8, ballykdy, 21, Burlingham, 15 (gloves), Daniel M Ernst, 18, Focus and Blur, 15 (coat), Golden Pixels LLC, 25, Gorodenkoff, 9, ittipon, 15 (otoscope, stethoscope, rubber hammer), Madlen, 15 (face mask), Milkovasa, 16, Monkey Business Images, 20, Pixel-Shot, 6, 23, Rido, 19, Rob Byron, Cover, Rocketclips, Inc., 7, 11, 17, StockLite, 1, Tyler Olson, 12, YAKOBCHUK VIACHESLAV, 5, 13; Wikimedia: Elliot & Fry, 28

Editorial Credits
Editor: Carrie Sheely; Designer: Kyle Grenz; Media Researcher: Jo Miller; Production Specialist: Kathy McColley

All internet sites appearing in back matter were available and accurate when this book was sent to press.

Printed and bound in China. 5870

Table of Contents

Words in **bold** are in the glossary.

What Is a Doctor?

Ouch! A boy falls. He cannot walk on his leg. It hurts too much. He goes to the doctor. The doctor checks the leg. He finds out the boy has a broken bone. The boy will wear a covering on his leg. It will keep the bone in place. Then the bone can heal.

Doctors help people who are hurt. They help people who are sick. Doctors also help people stay healthy. The people who go to a doctor are called **patients**.

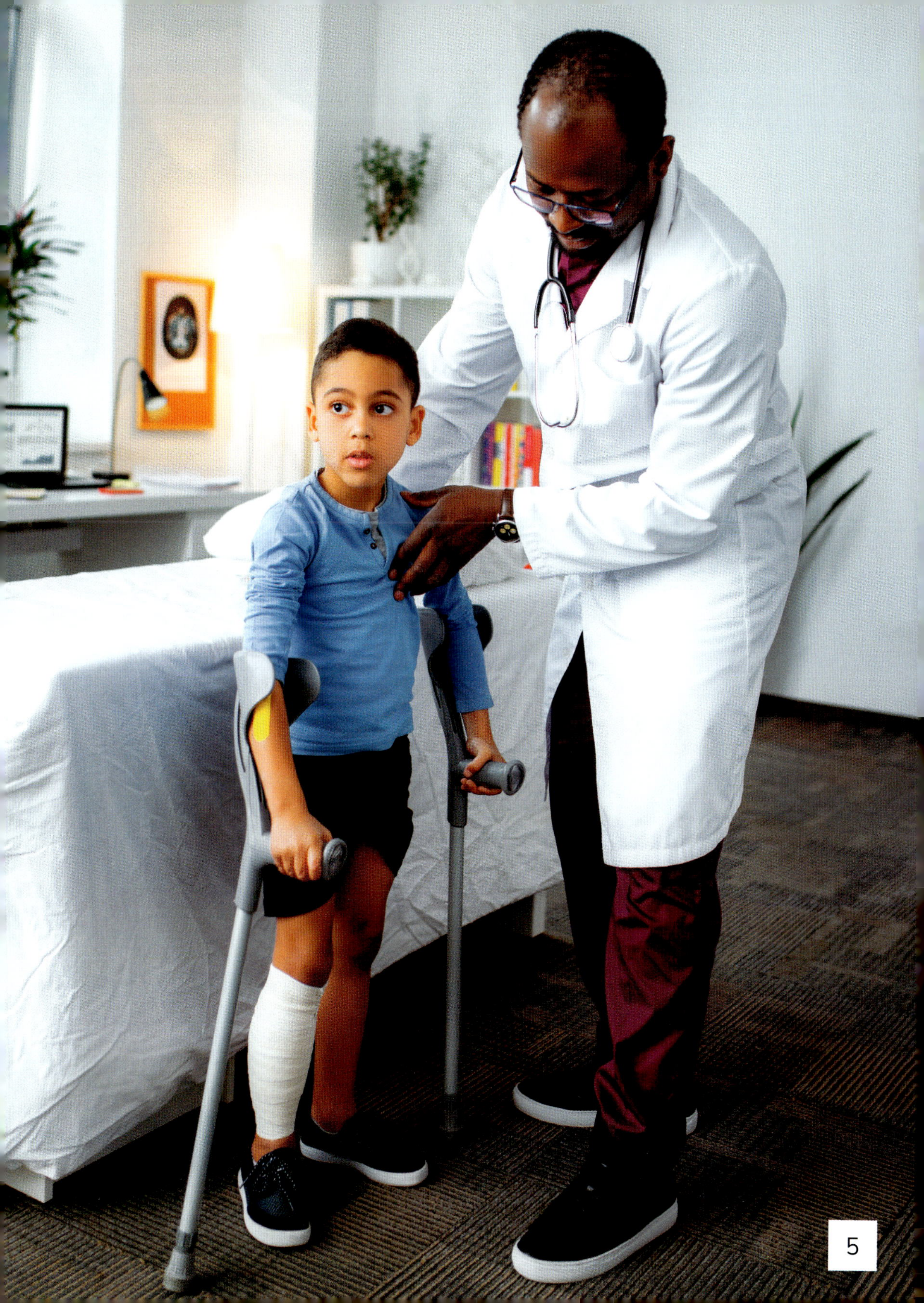

Types of Doctors

There are many kinds of doctors. Some help only babies and kids. You might go to one of these doctors when you get sick. You also might go to one for a **checkup**. At this visit, the doctor will make sure you are healthy and growing well.

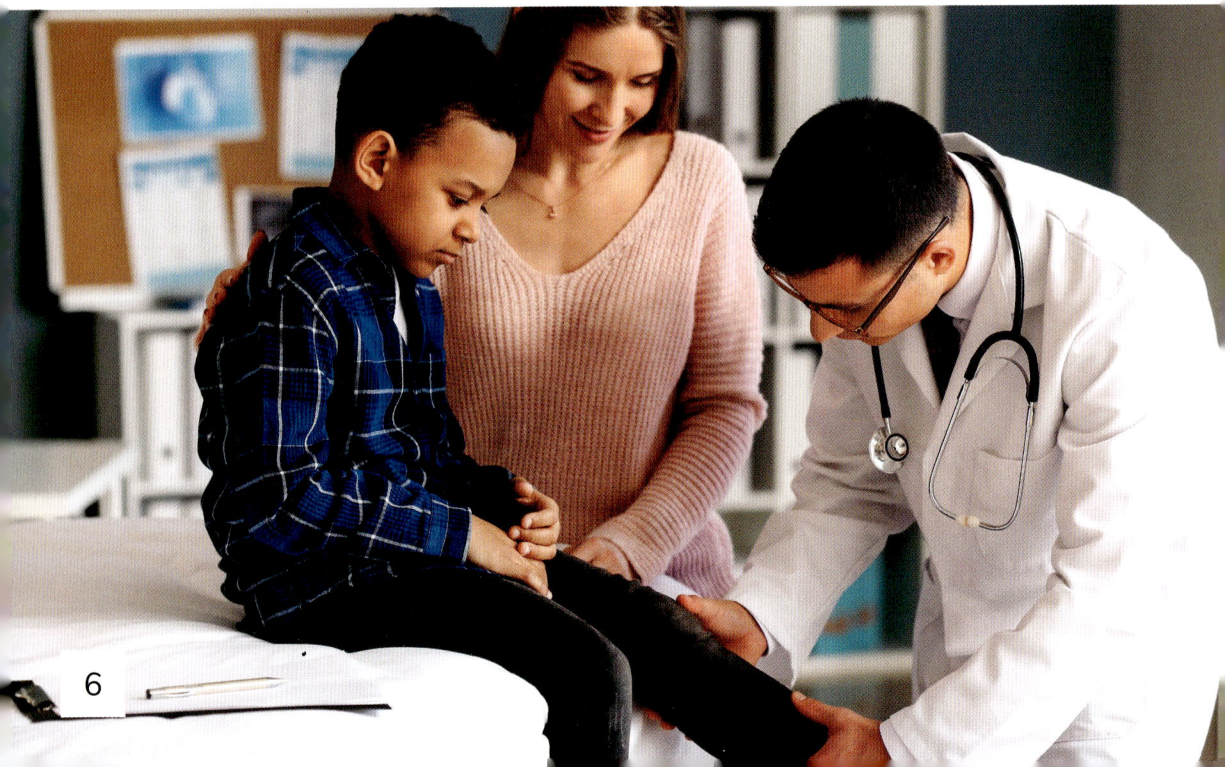

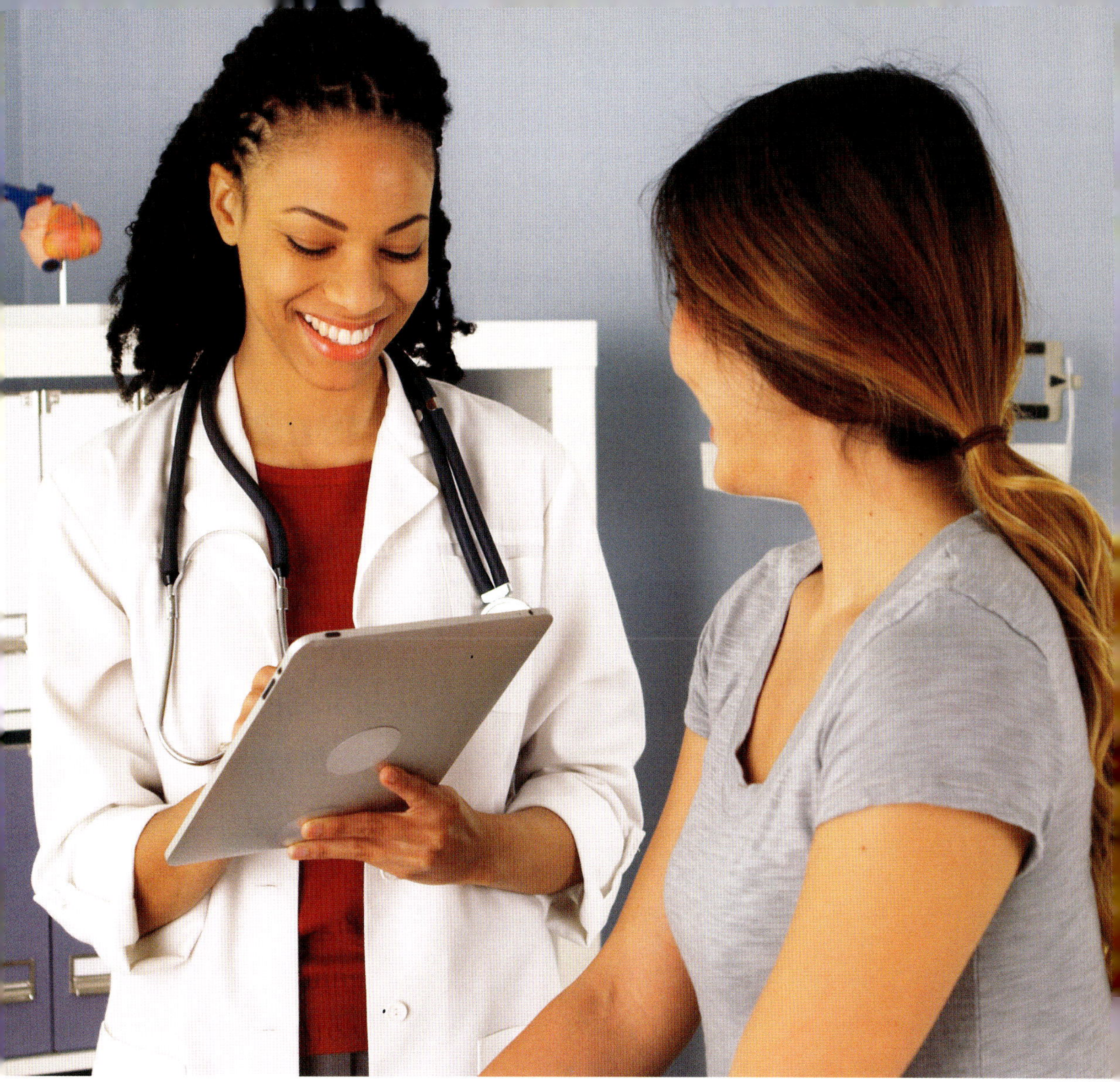

People of all ages go to family doctors. These doctors help people with many health problems. They give checkups too.

Other doctors give different care. Some help people with heart problems. Others help people with skin problems.

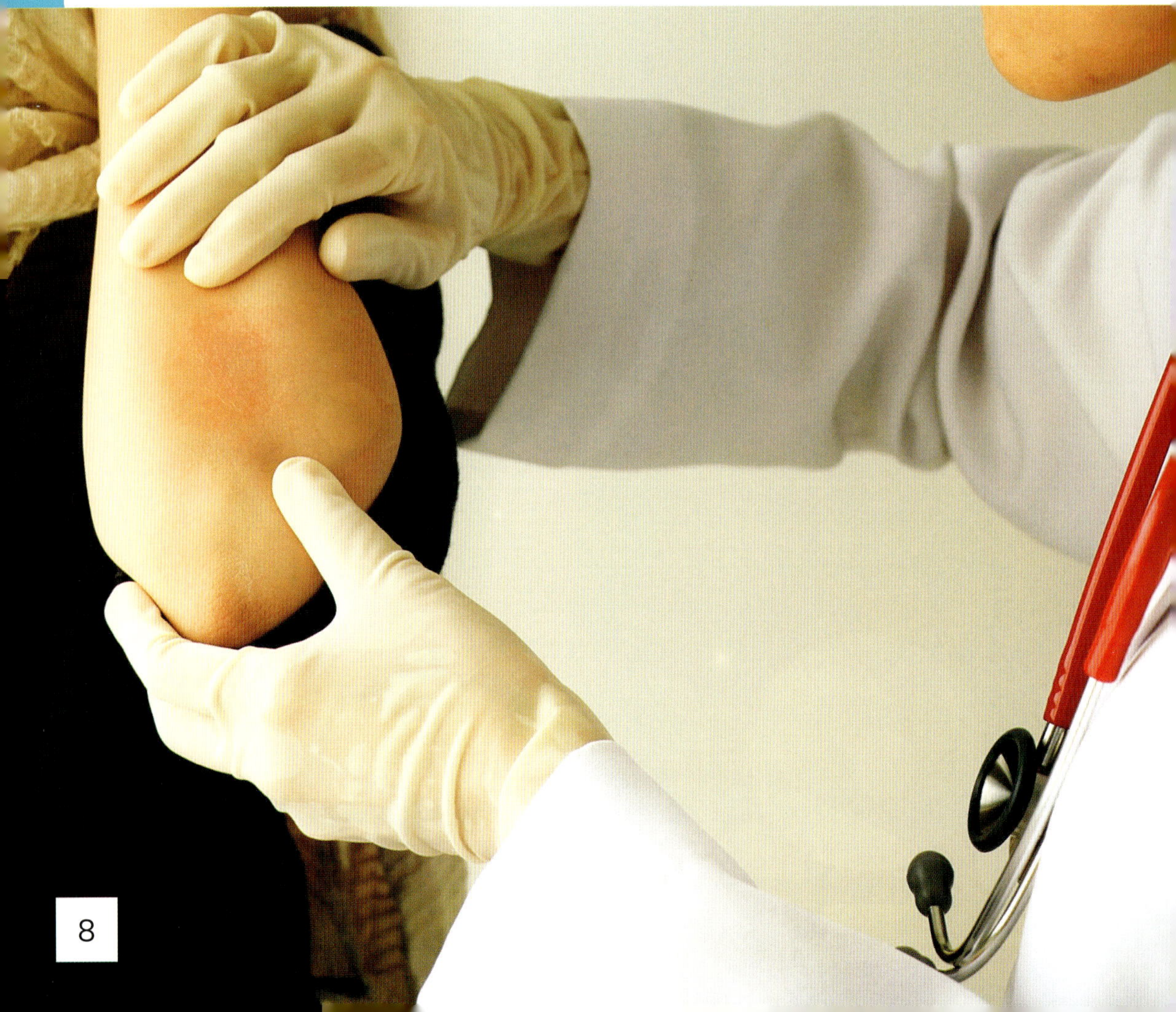

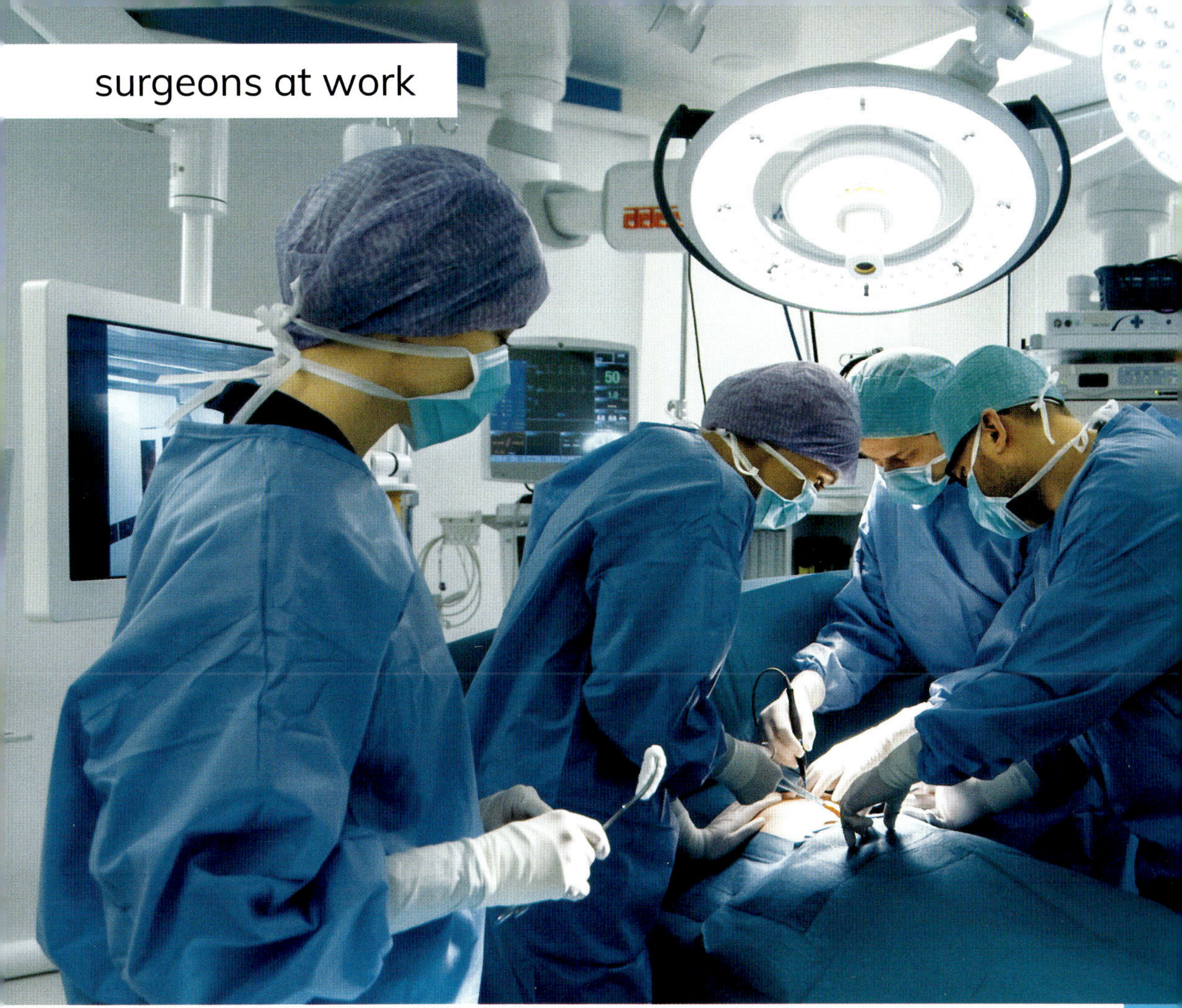

surgeons at work

Some doctors are trained to cut open the body. They are called surgeons. These doctors fix broken bones or body parts that are not healthy.

What Doctors Do

When you go to a doctor, you might see a nurse first. Doctors and nurses care for people together. Nurses check a person's height and weight. They do other tests too.

All the information gets saved in **records**. The doctor looks at the records. Nurses and doctors talk about the information.

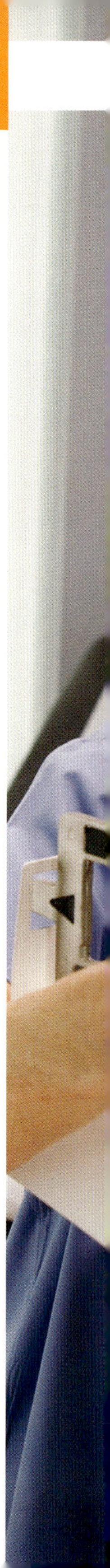

A nurse checks a patient's weight.

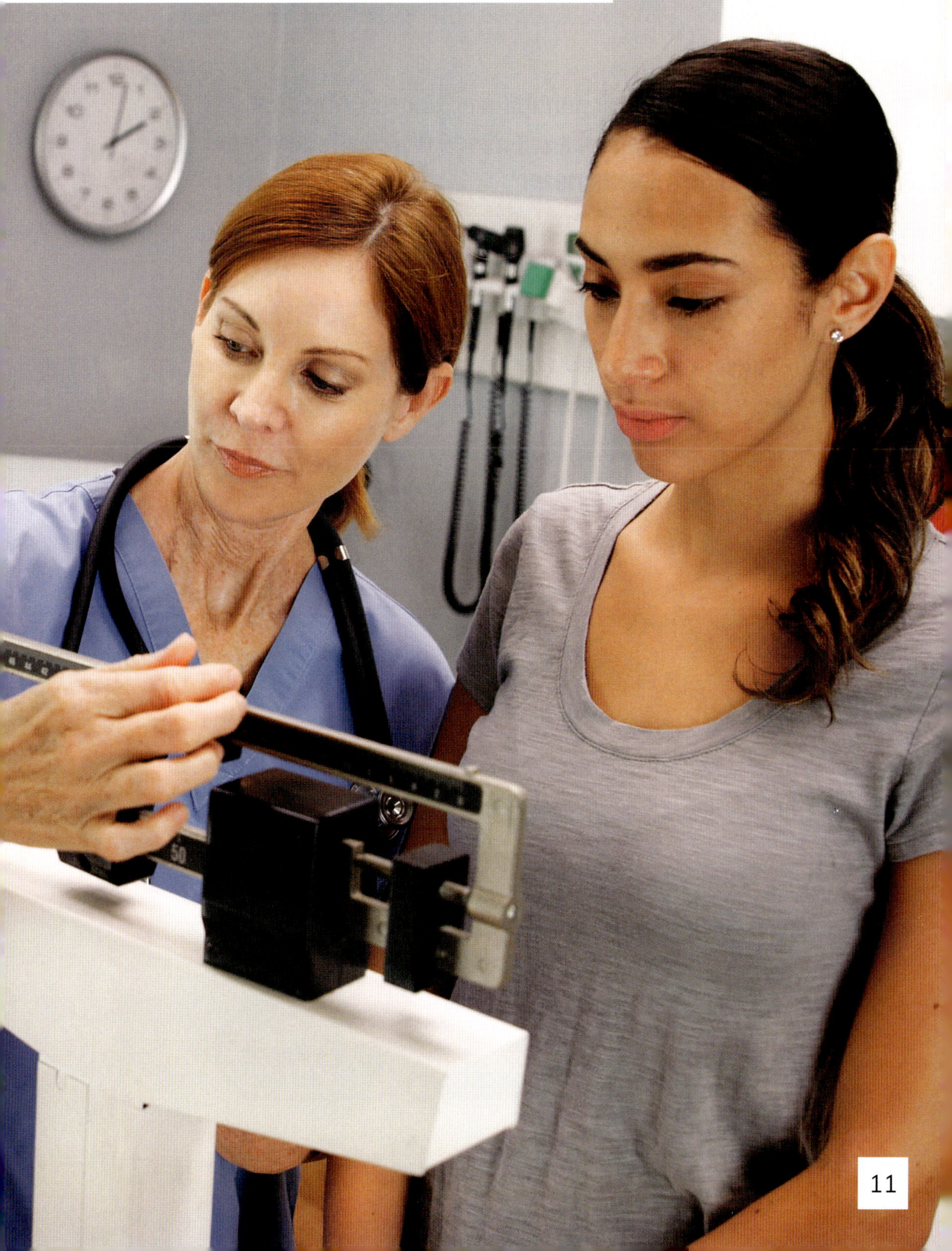

Next, the doctor checks the person's body. Before starting, a doctor might put on gloves. He or she might also wear a face mask. Gloves and masks can help keep people from getting sick. A doctor might wear a white coat too. It can help keep the doctor's other clothes clean.

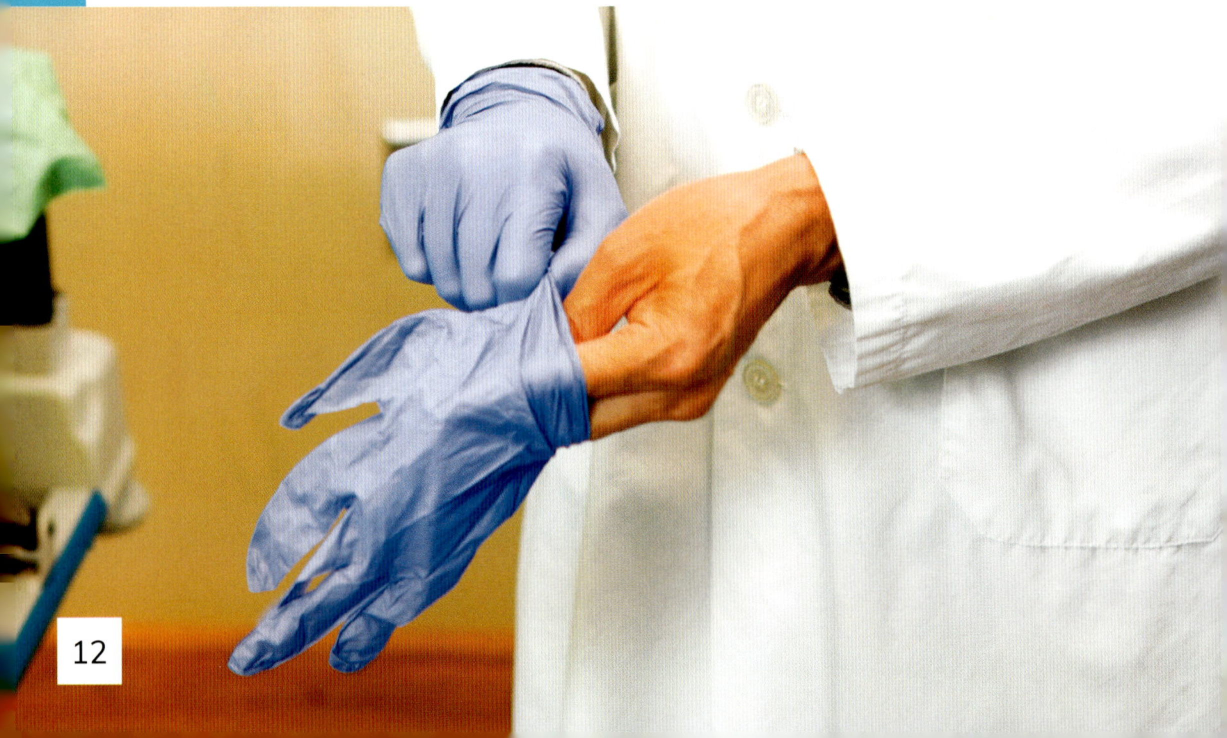

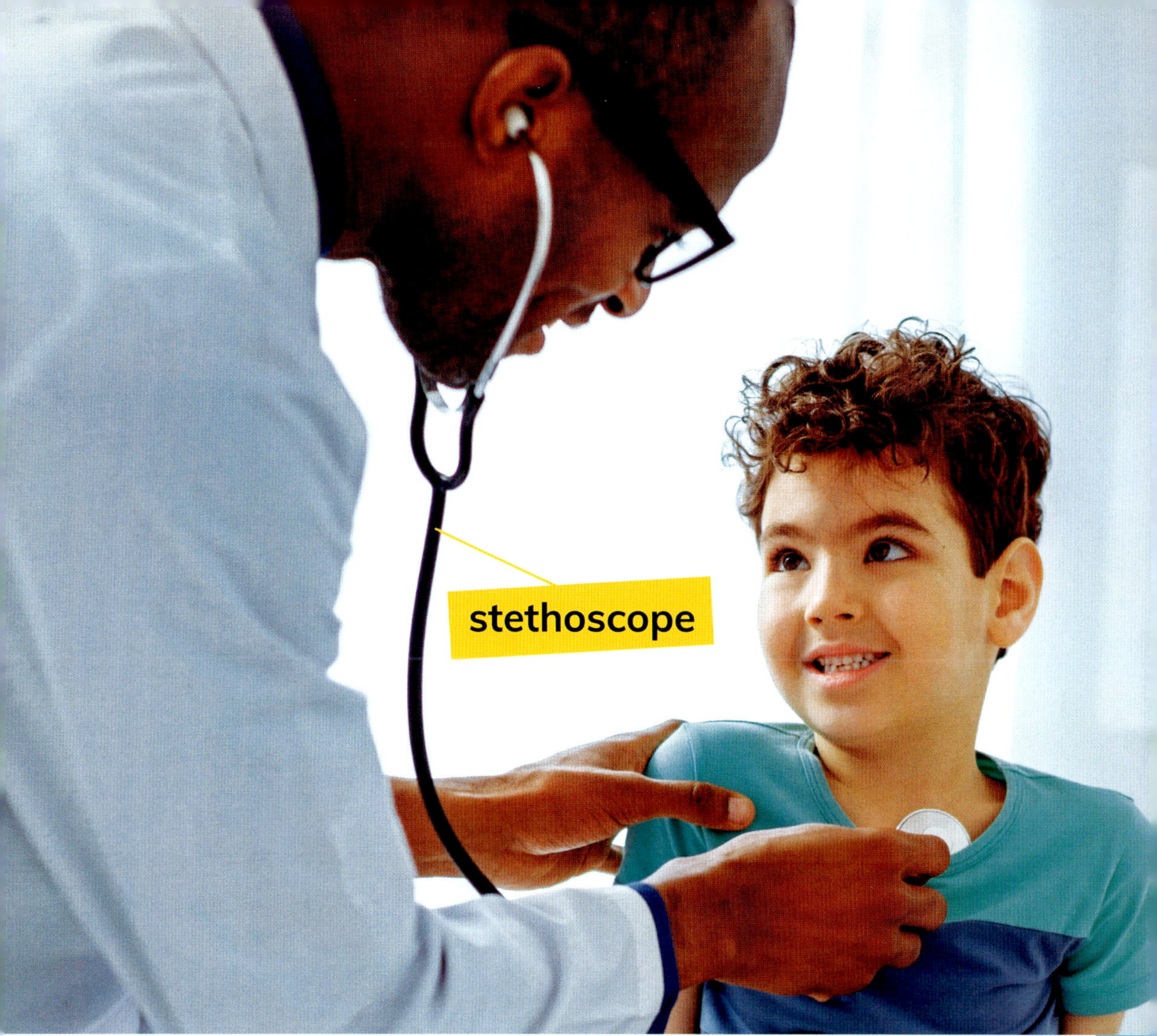

Doctors use many tools. They use a stethoscope. This tool lets the doctor hear a person's heartbeat and breathing.

Doctors also use tools to look closely at body parts. They see inside the ears, nose, and throat with an otoscope. Doctors use a different tool to check the eyes.

Doctors tap the knee with a rubber hammer. They see if the leg kicks up. This kick happens on its own. This test shows that the brain is working with the body like it should.

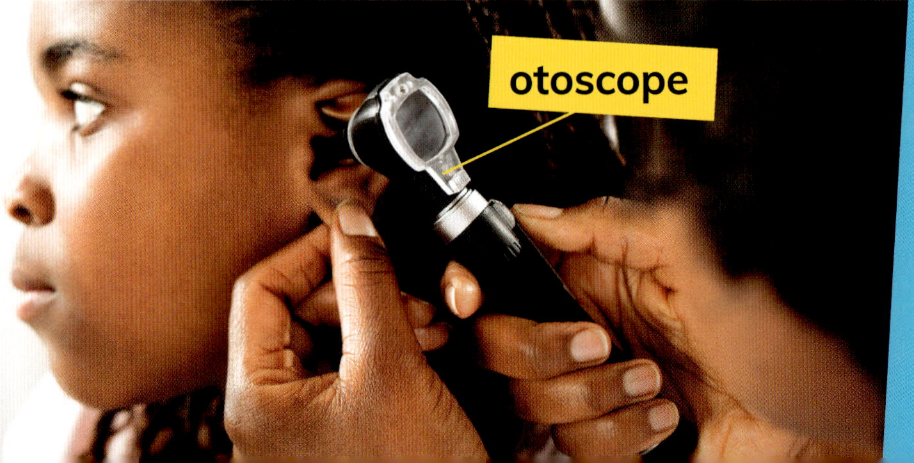

Tools Doctors Use

gloves

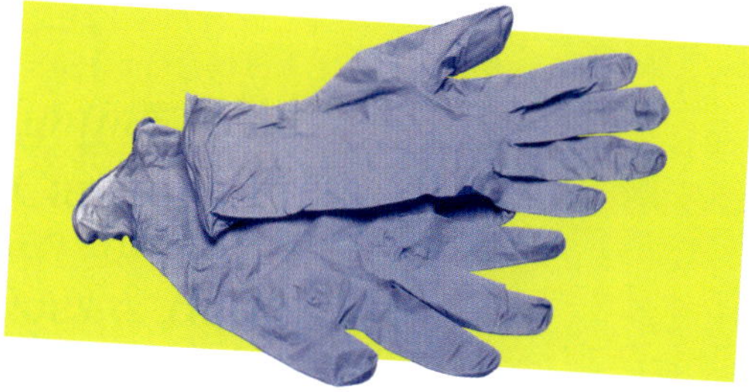

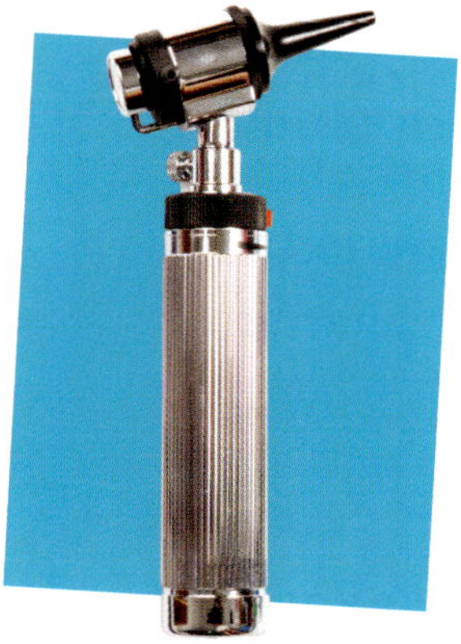

otoscope

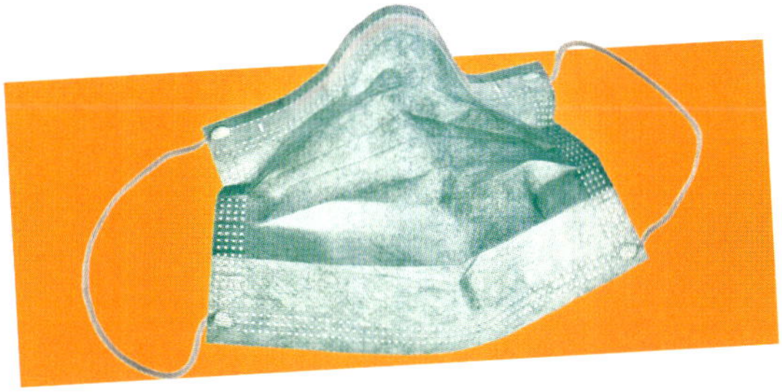

face mask

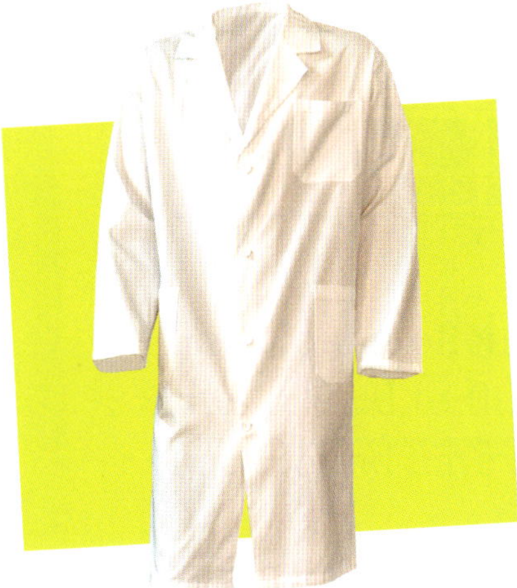

coat

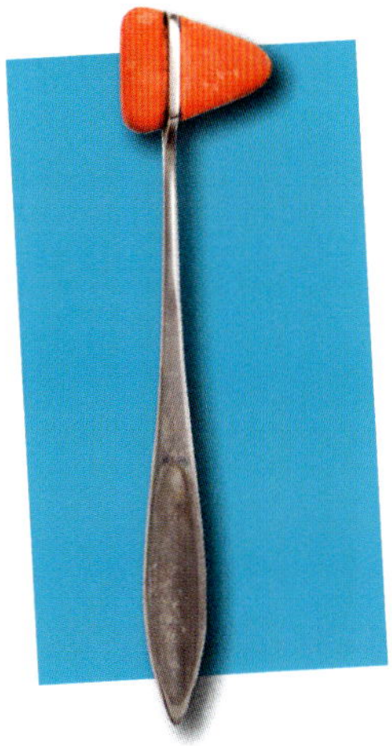

rubber hammer

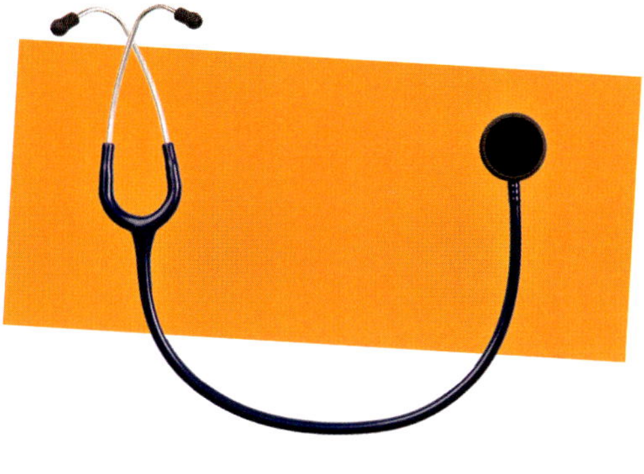

stethoscope

Sometimes people have signs of sickness. These signs are called **symptoms**. For example, a person's throat or ears might hurt. A person might have red bumps on his or her skin.

The doctor tries to find what is causing the signs. The doctor may need to get blood or other **samples**. **Lab** workers look closely at the samples. The doctor checks what they find.

A lab worker holds a blood sample.

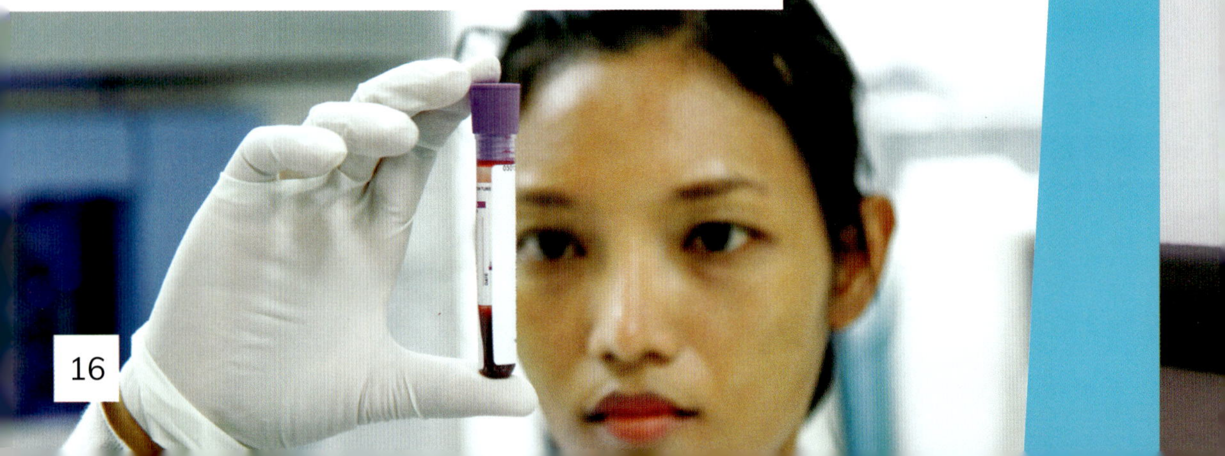

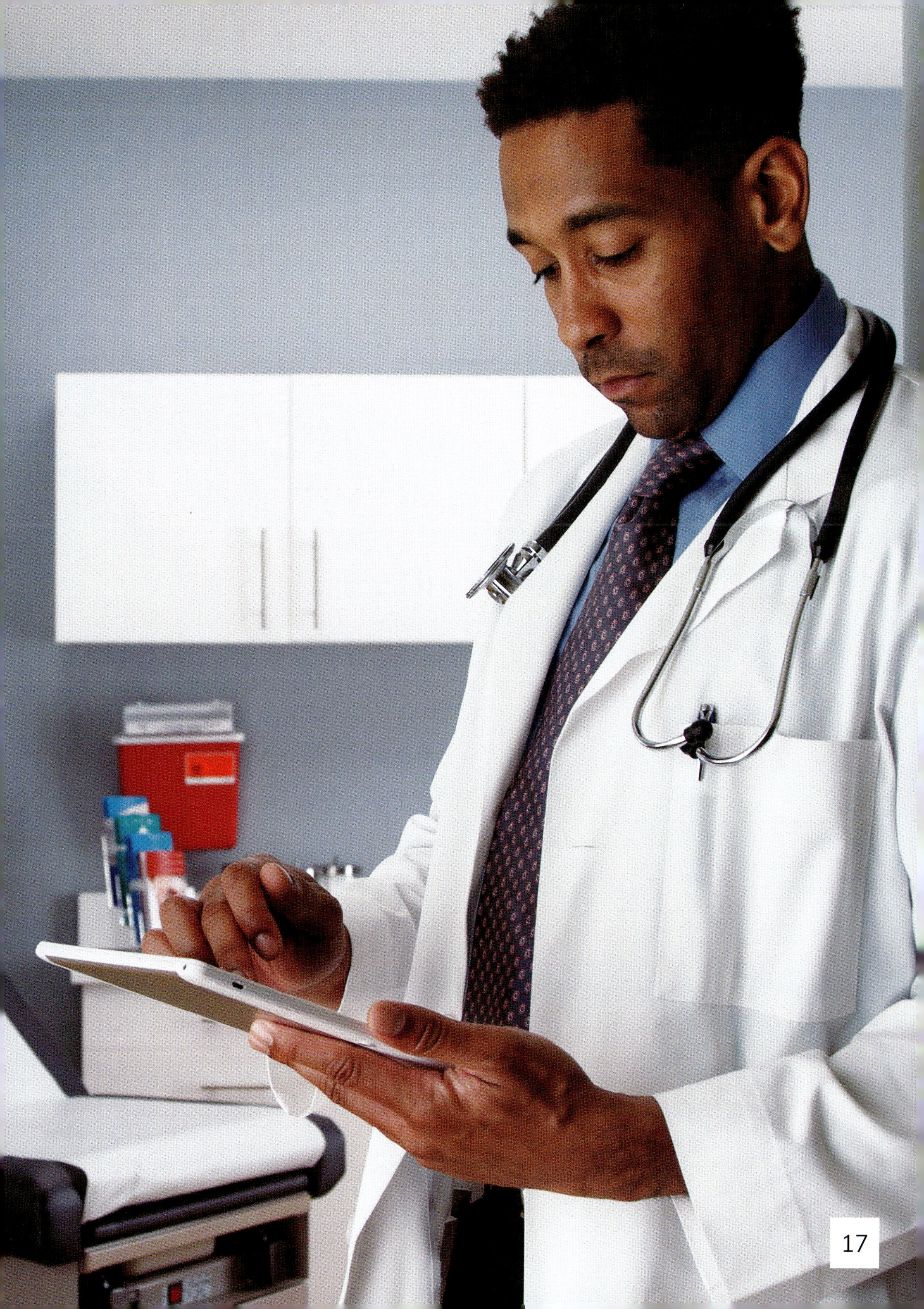

Doctors also ask questions to learn more. They may ask what a person usually eats. They might ask if people in the person's family have health problems. Doctors may need to talk to other doctors.

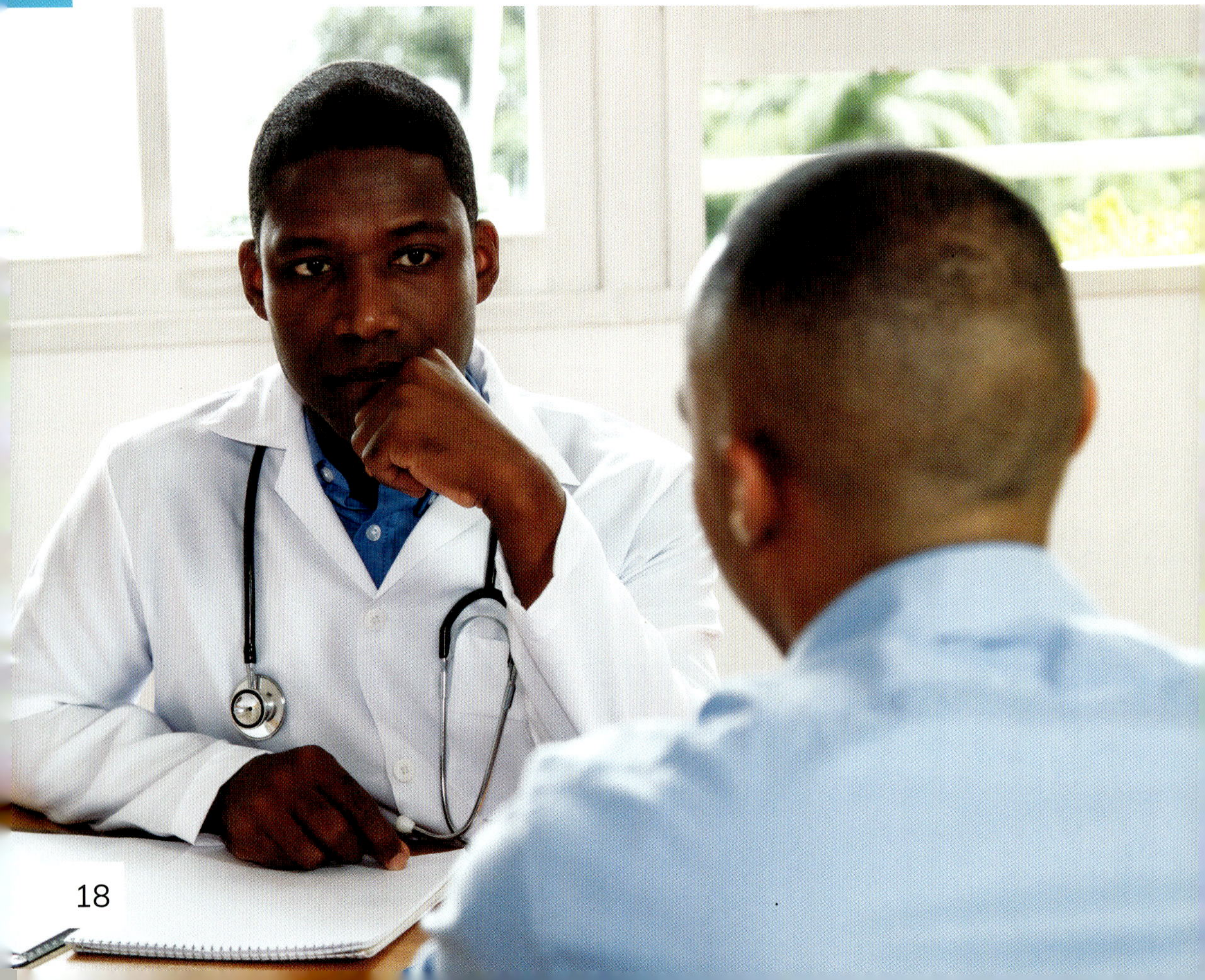

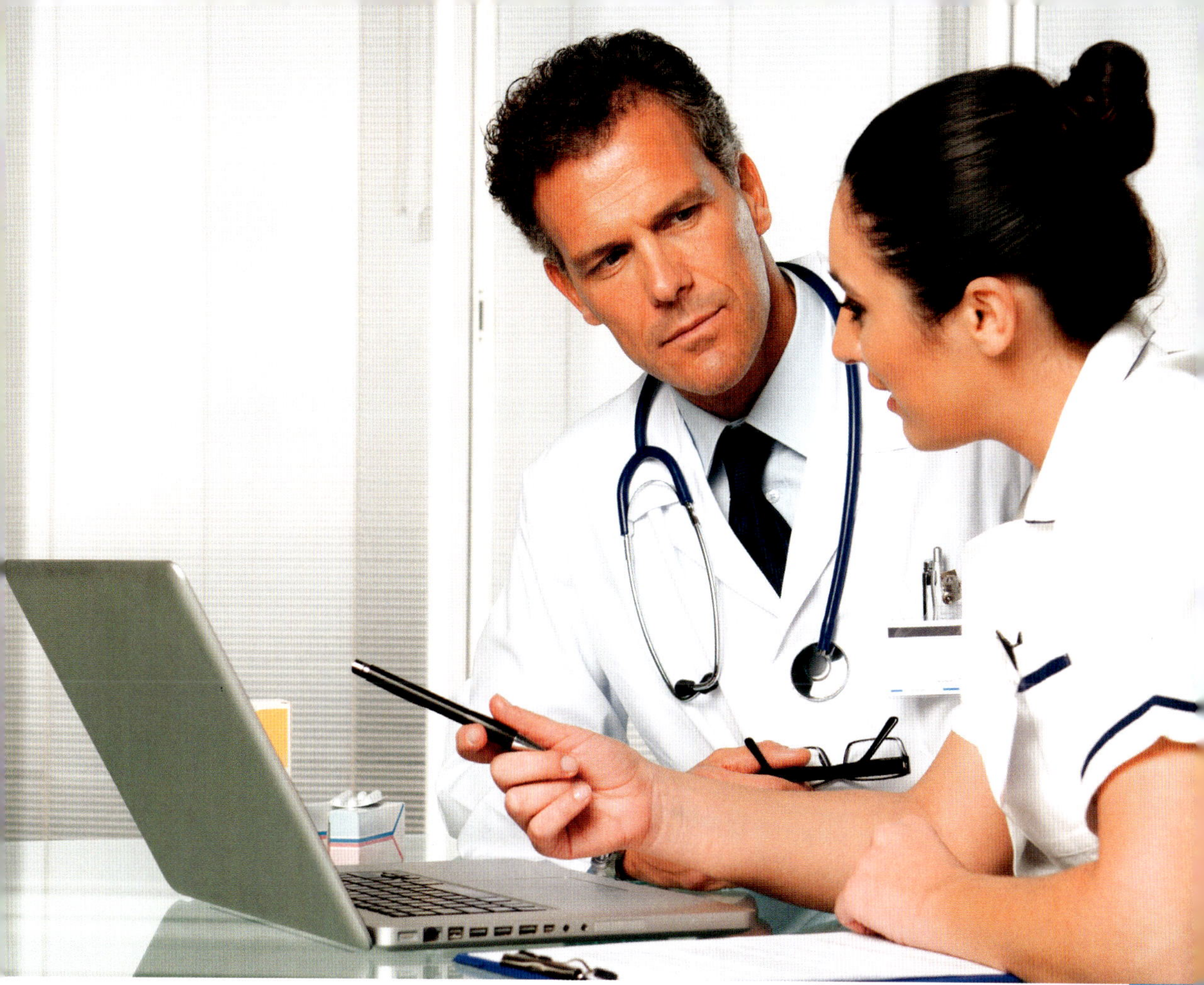

Doctors think about everything they learned. Often there is more than one way to explain the signs of sickness. Doctors decide which cause is most likely.

After finding a cause, a doctor tells the patient what it is. The doctor also says what **treatments** might help with the symptoms. This helps patients know how to get healthy.

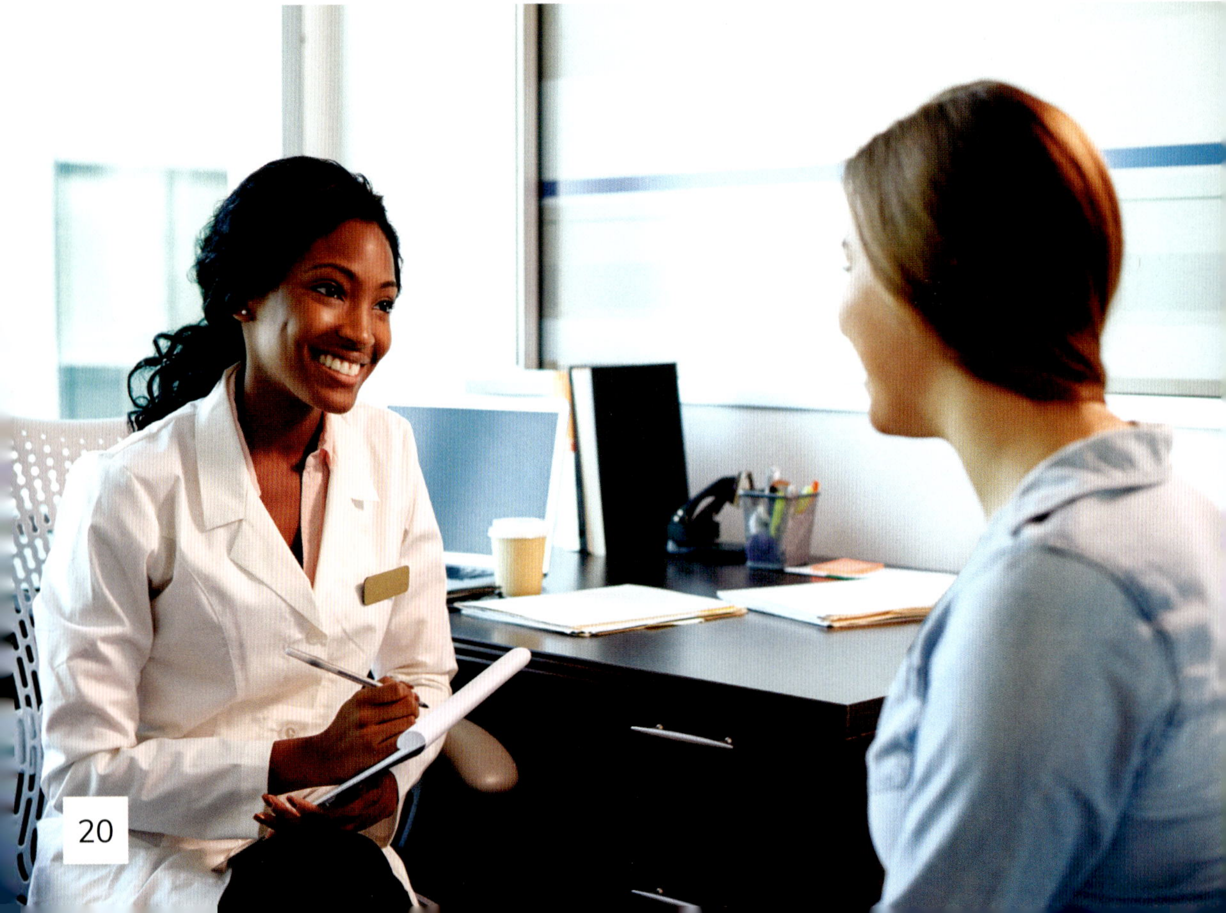

Sometimes small changes help. These could include getting more sleep or eating different foods. Other times doctors say taking **medicine** such as pills can help. Sometimes people need surgery.

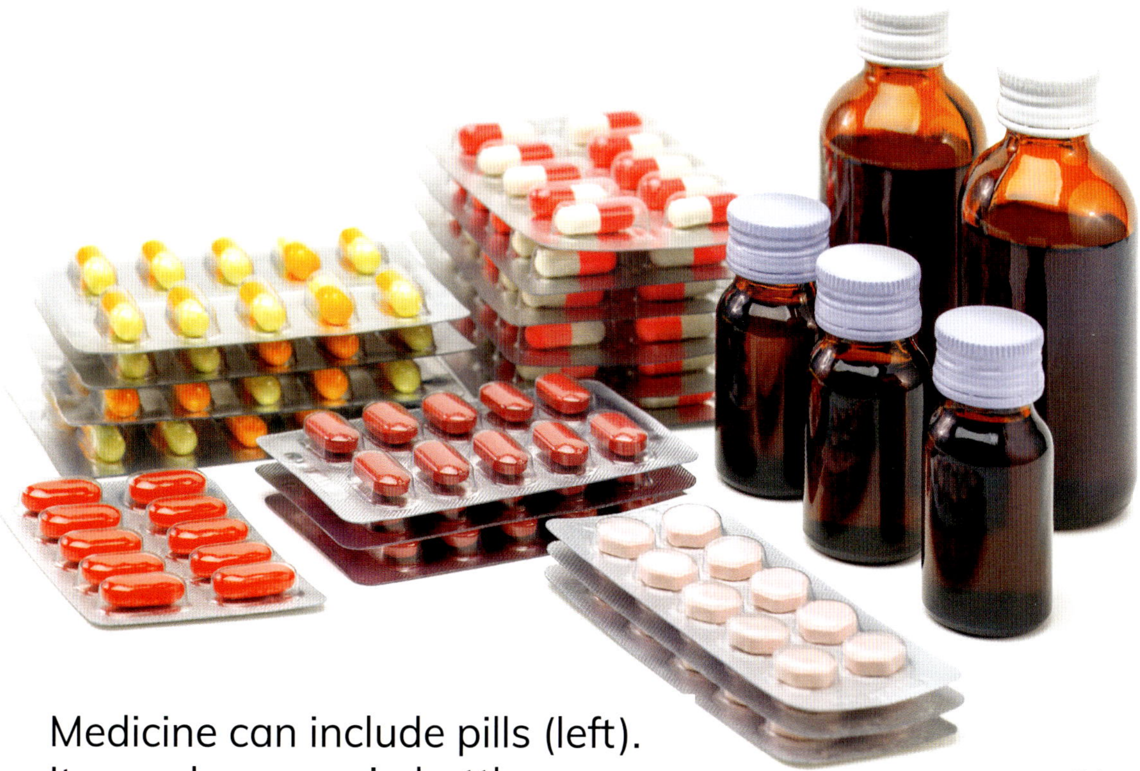

Medicine can include pills (left). It can also come in bottles.

Where Doctors Work

Some doctors work in clinics. They give checkups there. Doctors also treat common sicknesses there.

Other doctors work at hospitals. Doctors there help people with bigger problems. Most surgeries happen there.

Clinic and hospital doctors see many people a day. They work many hours. They may need to work overnight.

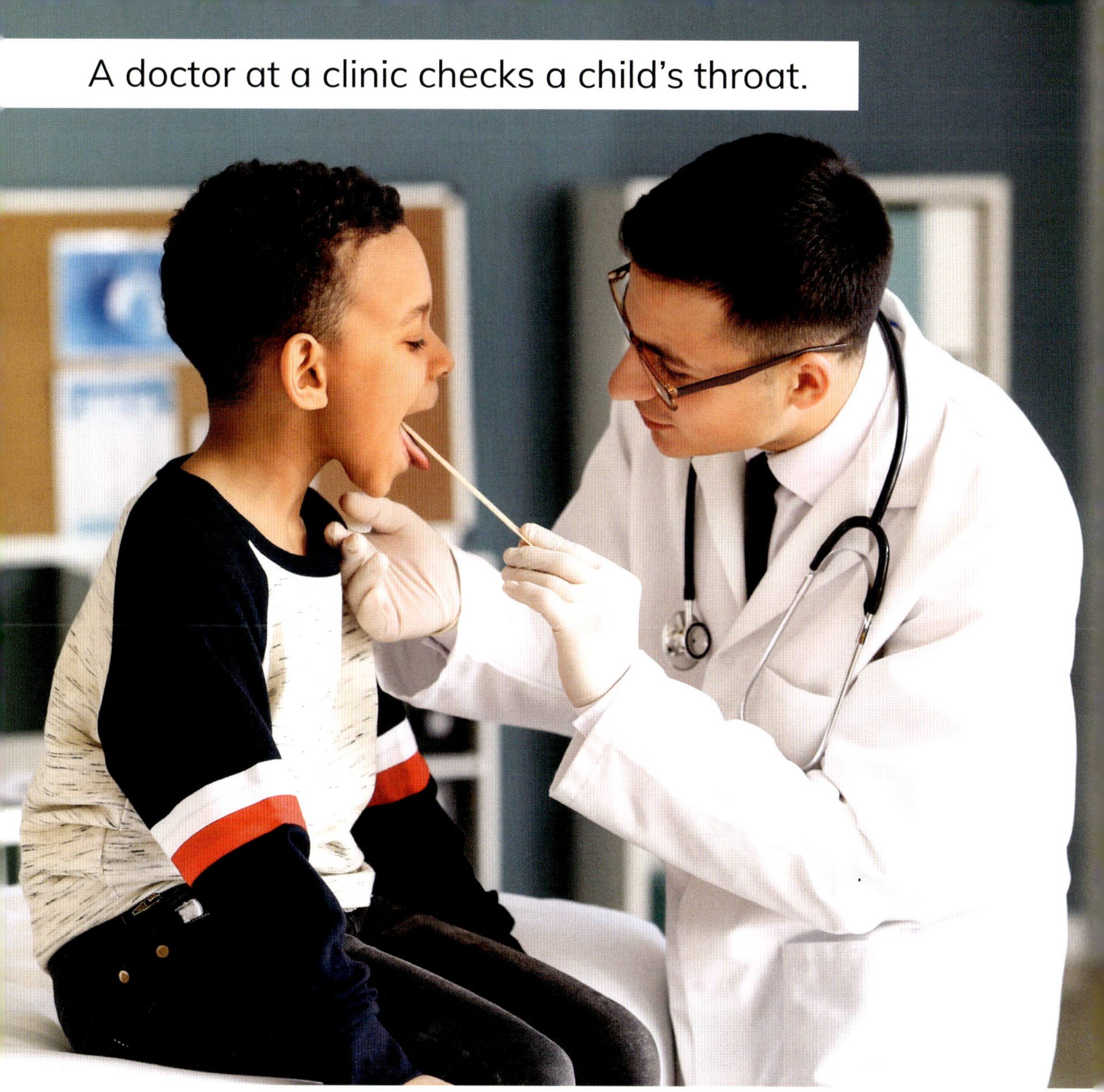

A doctor at a clinic checks a child's throat.

Other doctors work at teaching hospitals. These doctors teach students. The students are going to school to be doctors.

How to Become a Doctor

It takes a lot of training to become a doctor. People who want this job must first go to **college** for four years. Then they must pass a test to go to medical school. These schools are just for people who want to be doctors.

Medical school usually takes four years. Students take classes. They do tests and other hands-on work in labs. They spend the last two years of medical school working in clinics or hospitals.

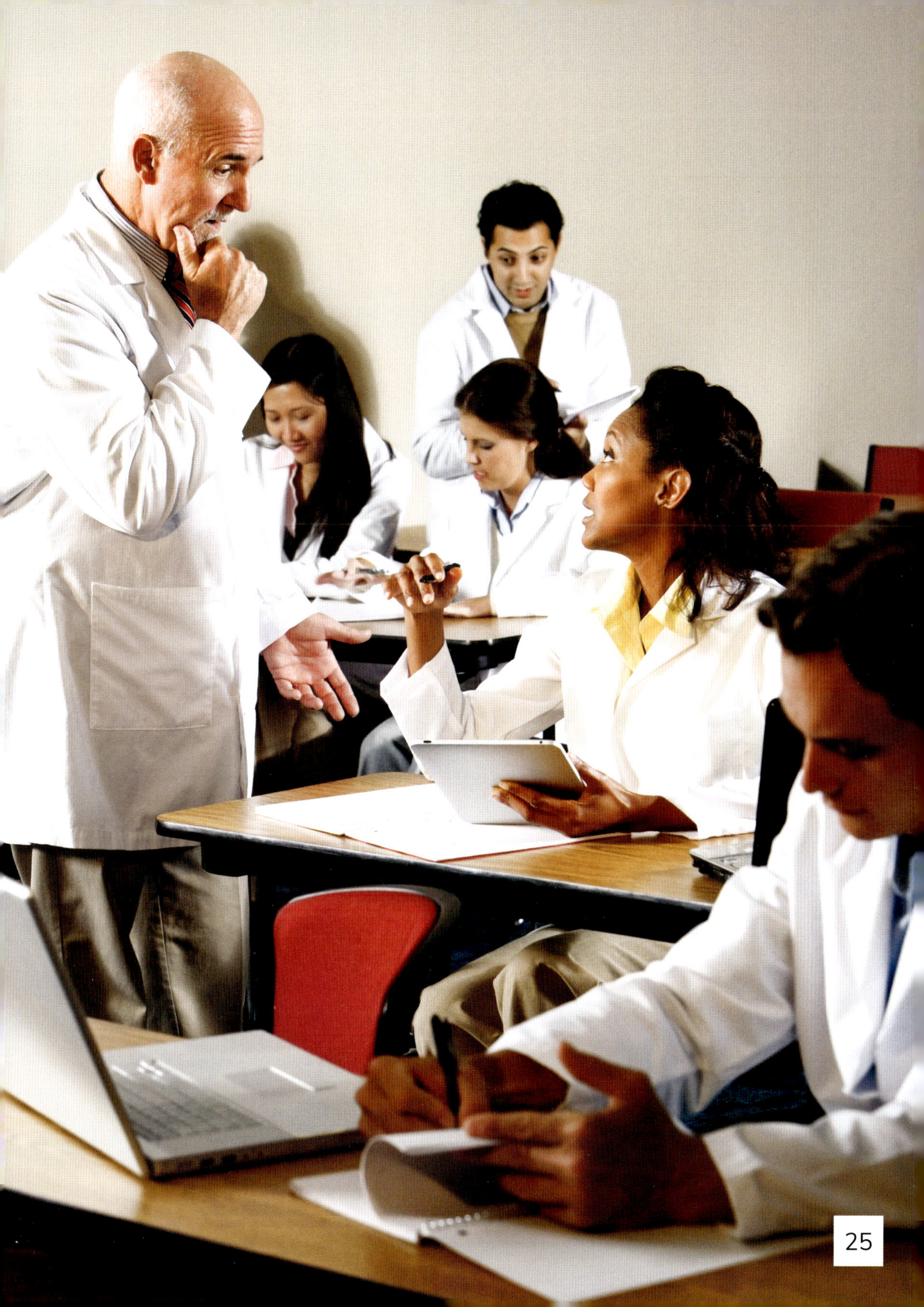

After medical school, students move on to residency training. This training usually takes at least three years. Students train in one kind of care. For example, they might train to become family doctors or surgeons. They work in hospitals and clinics. When their training is complete, they get a **license**. Then they can be doctors.

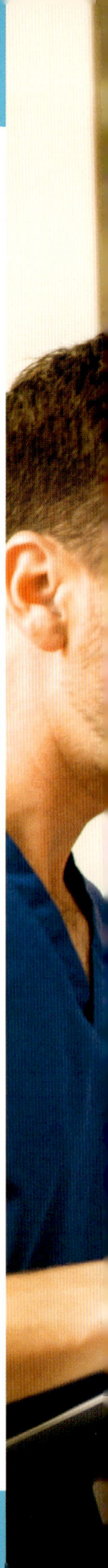

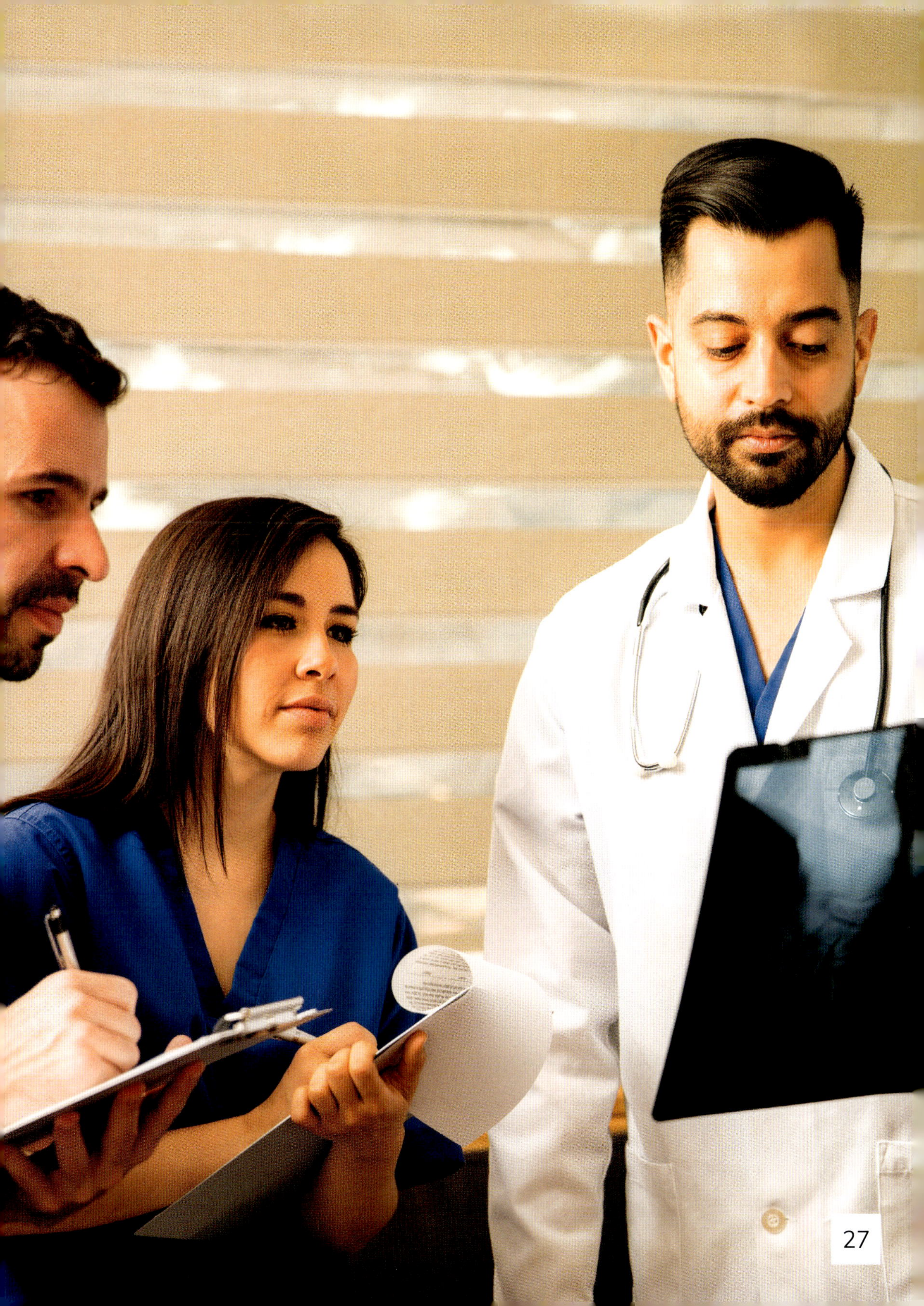

Famous Doctors

There are many famous doctors. Hippocrates was born about 460 BC in Greece. He studied the body. He understood that sicknesses had signs.

In 1849, Elizabeth Blackwell was the first woman to finish medical school in the United States. She opened her own clinic. Later, she opened a school for other women to become doctors.

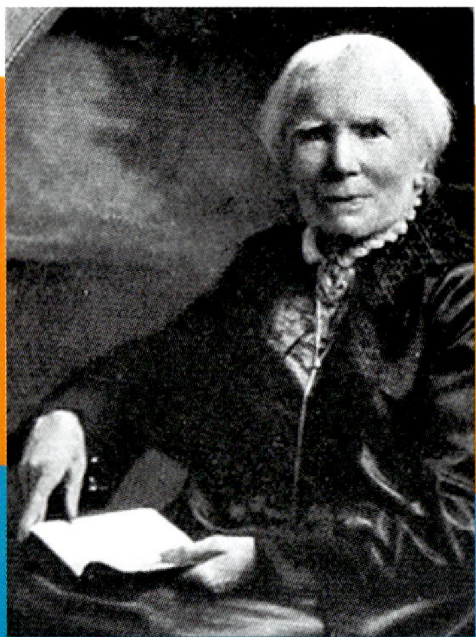

Elizabeth Blackwell

Fast Facts

- **What Doctors Do:**
  Doctors help sick and hurt people. They also help people stay healthy.

- **Where Doctors Work:**
  clinics, hospitals, teaching hospitals

- **Key Tools and Clothing:**
  coat, gloves, face mask, stethoscope, otoscope, rubber hammer

- **Education Needed:**
  college, medical school, residency training

- **Famous Doctors:**
  Hippocrates, Elizabeth Blackwell

Glossary

checkup (CHEK-uhp)—a visit to the doctor to be sure you are healthy

college (KOL-ij)—a school that students go to after high school

lab (LAB)—a place where experiments or tests are done

license (LYE-suhnss)—a document that officially makes it okay to do something

medicine (MED-uh-suhn)—a drug or other substance used to treat a sickness

patient (PAY-shunt)—a person who gets medical care

record (REK-urd)—a collection of facts

sample (SAM-puhl)—a small amount of something

symptom (SIMP-tuhm)—a sign that shows a person is sick or has a health problem

treatment (TREET-muhnt)—a way to heal, cure, or control symptoms

Read More

Hoena, Blake A. *The Doctor's Office: A 4D Book.* North Mankato, MN: Capstone Press, 2018.

King, Aven. *A Doctor's Tools.* New York: PowerKids Press, 2016.

Liebman, Daniel. *I Want to Be a Doctor.* Ontario, Canada: Firefly Books, 2018.

Internet Sites

Elizabeth Blackwell
https://www.womenshistory.org/education-resources/biographies/elizabeth-blackwell

Going to the Doctor
https://kidshealth.org/en/kids/going-to-dr.html

Just for Kids: Going to the Doctor
http://www.healthcommunities.com/just-for-kids/children/doctor-visit.shtml

Index